Lifting For Women:

Essential Exercise, Workout, Training and Dieting Guide to Build a Perfect Body and Get an Ideal Butt

By

Charles Maldonado

Table of Contents

Introduction

Chapter 1. Basic Principles of Lifting For Women

Chapter 2. Foods That Women Should Eat When Weight Lifting

Chapter 3. Various Exercising For Weight Lifting

Chapter 4. Training Plan

   Workout One

   Workout Two

   Workout Three

Chapter 5. Additional Tips

Conclusion

Thank You Page

Lifting For Women: Essential Exercise, Workout, Training and Dieting Guide to Build a Perfect Body and Get an Ideal Butt

By Charles Maldonado

© Copyright 2015 Charles Maldonado

Reproduction or translation of any part of this work beyond that permitted by section 107 or 108 of the 1976 United States Copyright Act without permission of the copyright owner is unlawful. Requests for permission or further information should be addressed to the author.

This publication is designed to provide accurate and authoritative information in regard to the subject matter covered. This work is sold with the understanding that the publisher is not engaged in rendering legal, accounting, or other professional services. If legal advice or other expert assistance is required, the services of a competent professional person should be sought.

First Published, 2015

Printed in the United States of America

Introduction

Lifting has been a way to keep people strong and it also helps in boosting their overall health. Lifting used to be only for the men, but nowadays more and more women are growing to love the concept of lifting and weight lifting contests for women are being held worldwide. There is also a way for women to lift weights and not get all that bulky which would depend on what they are taking while they lifting weights.

Muscles were made to be utilized well especially in making people move and be able to perform various physical activities throughout the day. When a person is lifting, she will be able to work both her upper and lower body. Lifting also requires optimum health because it requires your body to become very well-coordinated in order to lift properly. If lifting is not done correctly, it can cause problems in the joints and muscles. A person should also rest after a day of strenuous lifting and physical exercises.

People say that lifting is not for everyone, but it does require a lot of training and proper diet for you to be able to perform better when lifting. In this book, you will be able to read about the basic principles of lifting, what types of food you need to eat, what are the different exercises you can do to improve your lifting ability, how many times you need to exercise per week, how long you need to exercise, how your training should look like, and you will also be introduced to the training plan is recommended for lifting. You will have a better view on what training should be and what is to love about it. It is not only for men, but it has become popular as well. If you are interested in lifting, this book will make you realize why you should pursue your idea of starting to weight lift. It can also have different benefits to the body because you will not be following a certain diet, it will also help in making your body physically stronger and healthier.

After you have finished reading this book, you will have a head start in the world of lifting and what you can do to be able to perform it correctly. You will have a training plan that you can follow so that you will not be lost when you are getting started with lifting.

Chapter 1. Basic Principles of Lifting For Women

Principle one – Limiting factor

The exercise is more effective in the certain body part that is being trained if that body part is the one that becomes the limiting factor in the performance of that exercise while the other criteria is being overlooked. If during deadlifts your grip is already giving up, then the chain of your back will not become stimulated and the deadlifts won't become the best way to train your lower body. In the same way when you are performing a pull-up, your triceps and your lower chest are the most active, but both of them will not put a limit when you are doing a pull-up. This is the reason why pull-ups are not considered to be the most effective when it comes to training these body parts. The unstable exercises are removed from the exercise menu of the body builder by the criterion. When you stand on a surface that is unstable your balance will be challenged and also the muscles that work together to keep you stable which are the limiting factors in the exercise that you are performing. This principle is also applied when an unstable object is used as weight.

Principle Two – Being compounded

This is the most superior among exercises when it comes to exercises that are isolated, but the exercise should be able to fulfill the needs of the other body parts. If you are able to train three muscles all at one time, then what's the point of training them separately? The effect of compound exercises in your body is more hormonal, neurological, and cardiorespiratory compared what isolated exercises can do. Compound exercises add up to more than what isolated exercise parts can sum up to this means that the person who performs a lot of bench press is better than someone who does skull crushers and flys. Compound workouts also let the external force be spread in other joints of the body and this is good for the strength and health of the joints. In other words, it is a way to make your move more naturally and they are able to also target the isolated parts of your body.

Principle Three – Range of motion

An exercise is better if it's done in a full range of motion. It has been proven that when lifting with a full range of motion, is better than doing a range of motion that is only partial if you want to build strength. There was a study that tried to measure the size and there is a proven significance. One full exercise that is done with a full range of motion is better than doing partial ranges of motion in different parts of the full range of motion. This means that doing a bench press with a full range of motion is much better than doing only partial range of motion in the top, middle, and bottom positions combined. Doing a full range of motion will definitely increase the mobility of the movement pattern and it will also increase the length of the muscles which is more effective compared to stretching. Doing partial squats will not give full training to the back, but it will only be good for quad training and a little bit for the spinal erectors. And the when training in a full range of motion, it is better for your nervous system and your joints because you do not need a lot of weight. This means that if you are using lesser weights, but you are performing in a full range of motion, you will get a better exercise.

Principle Four- Stress distribution in the tissues

If the stress of an exercise is applied on the structures that are targeted, and there is less stress placed on the sides, the exercise will be better. Many sources give principles to the distribution of stress to the tissues which includes studying the EMG activity, compound movements against isolation, chain movements that are closed against open, and free weight movements against machine exercises. Specific exercises should be able to maximally stimulate muscles and also target the tendon because they are needed to adapt to be able to allow maximum growth of the muscles. Cardiovascular health, tendon strength, and bone density can handle themselves if you are doing compound exercises with high-intensity so you don't need worry about focusing on your muscles only. Your body is not built to perform exercises that are done behind your body so must eliminate front raises, dips, presses behind the neck, and your side behind the body exercises. The role of your core is to make the spine stable. Flexion is a spinal that is not really needed when body building. You should always keep your back flat because a position that is anatomical is mostly the best position for transferring force, activating the core, and shearing forces for the spine. If an exercise forces a specific movement pattern in your body, it will not be good for the criteria. This means that dumbbells are better than using barbells, but they are better than machines. Tissue stress distribution from free weights is more acceptable compared to machines.

Principle Five – Contraction that is dynamic

Exercises which have a portion of concentric and eccentric exercises are far better than exercises that are only eccentric, concentric, and isometric. There is a study showing that muscle mass located in the cross-sectional area is an evidence of this concept. Movements that are considered as dynamic contractions are easier on your joints which will let more production of force while in the concentric phase.

Principle Six – Resistance curve is equal to strength curve

The better the exercise will become if the person who is a healthy trainer has a strength curve that is approximated by the resistance curve that is closer. If the curve strength and the resistance of an exercise don't match, there will be muscles during the lift that will not become stimulated. The exercise will be able to develop the muscles that are used in the movement in a manner that is structurally balanced. A healthy trainer pertains to you not failing to do the deadlifts properly because failing to do a deadlift is caused by poor structural balance. If you fail repeatedly, this might mean that you have weak glutes that are disproportioned keeping you from performing the deadlift correctly.

Principle Seven – Micro Loadability

The exercise is better if the resistance can be determined more precisely. The exercises that are considered best for mass-building extend themselves to small increments of load and high loads. Ideally, lifters want to do exercises that increase max weights of the weights that are being used, but small steps need to be taken to maximize them. Maximum or absolute is considered to be a factor that is limiting to bodyweight exercises. Handstand push-ups are better than presses done overhead respecting the kinetic chain, but they are much worse than presses done overhead with absolute loading. You can add more resistance as you are able to perform more exercises at once because incremental can be a limiting factor for a lot of exercises. There are fixed increments found in machines and most of the gyms only have weights available that only increase Five pounds each time. You can only load small plate's times Two in barbells because you cannot use lopsided bars. Even if beginners and intermediates can progress with different increases, the load that is being added incrementally should only be within the percentage of the weight that is working so it does not have to be five to ten pound increments. Five pounds might be a good idea for doing squats, but it is bad for the isolation work of your shoulders.

Chapter 2. Foods That Women Should Eat When Weight Lifting

Women should eat lean meat because they will be able to make up for your protein requirements when weight lifting. Protein is needed by all athletes to build stronger muscles. There can be a lot of sources of protein, but some are better than others. Buying lean meats mean that you get them without the fat in groceries. Best way to cook this healthily is by grilling it so that any extra fat will drip away before you eat it. Chicken and turkey don't contain as much iron as red meat, but they can be cooked in more dishes and less problems are caused by chicken and turkey compared to red meat. Do not buy composite slices that might contain a lot of fat. Still go for lean chicken and turkey meat. The amino acid that is present tin lean meat can help repair and build muscles.

Low-fat dairy products like cheeses and yogurt have both calcium and protein, but stay away from cheese that contain a lot of fat. If you only eat Brie or blue cheese occasionally, that is fine. If you need to observe the low-calorie diet, you need to be careful of sweetened and low fat yogurt because they have more sugar. Dairy products have amino acid and calcium that are good for maintaining and rebuilding muscles. The low-fat ones can limit saturated fat and the consumption of cholesterol. Fish and seafood like salmon and sardines are also called oily fish which have a lot of omega-3 fats which are very important for the body's function. They can also benefit the heart by being an anti-inflammatory fat, learning mood, and other brain functions. Fish oils which contain omega-3 can also help you to lose weight. Fish supplements have become very popular with body builders during the phase of weight loss for targeting low body fat.

Shrimp and crabs contain a lot of cholesterol, but they won't raise blood cholesterol if they are only consumed moderately. Iodine is an important mineral that is present in seafood, this might become important parts when there is not much iodine in food. Seafood and fish give important omega-3, iodine, and polyunsaturated fats. Mono and Polyunsaturated fats and oils are important for some critical functions in the body. The vegetables that contain monounsaturated and polyunsaturated fat can improve the reading of the cholesterol in blood and also the high-density cholesterol (HDL) that us good for protecting the heart against diseases. Seeds and nuts are believed to contain a lot of omega-6 oils and monounsaturated oils which are considered the vegetable version of omega-3 fats. Cauliflower and sunflower are vegetable oils which mostly contain polyunsaturated omega-6 fats. Monounsaturated fats can be found in seeds, nuts, olives, and in other cuts of meat. Most of the vegetable oils have enough amount of monounsaturated oils except for coconut oil and palm oil. Polyunsaturated fats can be found mostly in products coming from seeds like sunflower, safflower, canola and a lot of other nuts. Olive oil and peanut oil can be used when you are cooking salads.

The green leafy vegetables always play a role and they are lettuce, spinach, kale, cabbage, and broccoli. They all contain the vitamins and minerals such as magnesium, potassium, iron, and vitamin c. Carotenes are great for getting antioxidants and they also produce anticancer agents. If you consume this daily, it will promote your good health. Antioxidants give enough protection to our body against damage that is produced by high-intensity exercises and regular weight training. Green leafy vegetables that are nutrient-dense, give important nutrients if you are trying to lose weight. Vegetables that are red, purple, orange, and yellow like sweet potato, carrots, peppers, beetroot, eggplant, and red cabbage have a lot of antioxidants, flavonoids, carotenes, polyphenols, and anticancer factors. Eating these vegetables can help you withstand weight training and promote good health.

Blueberries, raspberries, strawberries, and blackberries all contain a high level of antioxidant. Persimmons have a lot of carotene which has lutein that is great for the eyes as people age. Bananas have a lot of potassium even if they contain a lot of sugar. You can always take this in moderation. Potassium is essential in making your blood pressure normal. Fruits are a good supply of protective nutrients and antioxidants. Carbohydrates found in fruits are important for keeping you energized when training to keep your immune system healthy. Beans have antioxidants, protein, fiber, potassium, calcium, and soluble fiber which are all very good for the keeping heart healthy. Nuts have fatty acids that are important. They also contain zinc, magnesium, protein, fiber, folate, B6, and iron. Brazil nuts have the most concentration of mineral selenium compared to other food. Almonds have the highest amount of calcium. Walnuts can be eaten if you want a rich source of omega-3 fats. Consumption of nuts is connected to lesser heart disease. Nuts have a wide variety of all the important vitamins, minerals, and nutrients that are all important for the health, immunity, and physical strength.

Chapter 3. Various Exercising For Weight Lifting

Plank and rotate

Start in a plank position while 2 5-poun dumbbells are in your hands. Keep your wrists stiff to be able to protect the joints. Your feet should be slightly wider than hip distance apart. Lift your left hand with the dumbbell towards the ceiling and your torso rotating. Your pelvis will start to rotate, but keep it balanced. Twist your torso back and your hand back on the floor and repeat the same steps with your right hand. Do this for 10 to 15 repetitions.

Squat and curl press

Stand with your feet hip width apart and holding a dumbbell in each hand. Keep your spine straight, start to squat down as low as you can and the weights should be near your heels. Your thighs should be parallel to the floor, but make sure your knees do not exceed your toes. Use force on your heel to get back to standing position and then do a bicep curl. Then extend your arms over your head for an overhead press. Lower both of your arms to your side to complete the repetition. Do this for 10 to 15 repetitions.

Circle and bend warm-up

Stand in a straight position with your feet hip width apart. If you have a weight ball, hold it with both hands using the handles on each side and lift it over your head put keep your knees soft. Lift your torso up and slowly stretch to the side and make a circular motion. Then bring both arms down to the floor and your knees slightly bent. Continue to circulate until you are back to the original position.

Do this for ten times and then reverse your rotation.

Shoulder shrug

Stand straight with your feet hip width apart. Holding five to fifteen pound dumbbells in each hand then slowly raise your shoulders high and count to 3 and then slowly lower one shoulder and then do this on the other side.

Do this for fifteen repetitions.

Bicep curls

Stand straight and put move your right leg slightly forward. You should be holding ten pound dumbbells in each hand. Bend your right arm towards your shoulder holding the weight. Put it back down beside you and then raise your left arm towards your shoulder.

Do two to three sets of fifteen repetitions.

How many times should weight lifting be done each week?

There's a lot of confusion when it comes to this one and people end up lifting weights too often to or too less. If you are just starting out, you can do two to three times per week and refrain from training the same muscle group in two consecutive days, but you can do weight lifting two days in a row just not with the same muscle groups.

The growth of the muscle tissues happen when your body is recovering. It is usually 24 to 48 hours when the muscles go through recuperation. You will notice that you are experiencing muscle soreness and this is when the body is underdoing muscle repair that have been torn. A good sleep is needed during this time because this is when the hormones of the body are working harder to make up for the stress in the muscles caused by weight training.

How long should you exercise?

Ideally, it should only be 30 to 60 minutes every workout session of heavy lifting depending on your fitness level.

Chapter 4. Training Plan

1st month

Workout number one and cardio for week one

Workout number two and cardio for week two

Workout number three and cardio for week three

Workout number one and cardio for week four

2nd month

Workout number two and cardio for week five

Workout number two and cardio for week six

Workout number three and cardio for week seven

Workout number two and cardio for week eight

3rd month

Workout number two and cardio for week nine

Workout number three and cardio for week ten

Workout number two and cardio for week eleven

Workout number one and cardio for week twelve

Cardio workout

For Monday, Wednesday, and Friday

You can do a treadmill interval by doing the following steps below for seven times in a span of 35 minutes

one minute with an incline of five and run at 4.5

two minutes with an incline of five and run at 5.0

three minutes with an incline of one and run at 5.5

Do 50-yard sprints, but do 30-second jogs in between sprints

For Tuesday and Thursday

You first need to warm-up for five minutes on a treadmill or stationary bike but only at low speed

one minute at level five with an rpm of 110

one minute at level seven with an rpm of 90

one minute at level nine with an rpm of 80

two minutes at level one with an rpm of 70

Do fifteen high jumps (wide)

fifteen quick squats

Do fifteen switch lunges on both legs

Twenty knee runs with both legs

Workout One

Monday

Superset

two sets of 15 leg extensions

two sets of 15 leg curls

Superset

four sets of 20 wide leg presses

four sets of 20 shoulder-width smith machine squats

Superset

four sets of 15 leg extensions

four sets of 15 narrow hack squat

Superset

four sets of 15 leg curls

four sets of 15 stiff legs

Tuesday

Superset

four sets of 12 side lateral raises

four sets of 15 one arm dumbbell shoulder presses

four sets of 15 lateral raises

five sets of incline presses

Superset

four sets of 15 pushdowns

four sets of 12 bench dips

Wednesday

five sets of wide-grip pulldowns

Superset

four sets of 15cg cable rows

four sets of 20 hyper extensions

Superset

Five sets of 15 preacher curls

five sets of 12 incline dumbbell curls

Thursday

Superset

two sets of 20 leg extensions

two sets of 20 leg curls

Do four reps in one circuit with no rest in between the moves. Rest for one minute after each round

Superset

ten high jumps (wide)

Jump as high as you can and do a deep squat for five seconds after every jump

fifteen switch lunges on both legs

ten bench step-up jumps on both legs

fifteen reverse lunges on both legs

ten gallop squats on both legs

Friday

four sets of 10 shoulder presses

four sets of 10 wide-grip pulldowns

Superset

four sets of 15 on each leg using the leg butt machine

four sets of 15 good mornings

five sets of 10 bench step-ups

Workout Two

Monday

Superset

four sets of twelve leg extensions

four sets of twelve weighed barbell of the reverse lunge

Superset

four sets of fifteen dumbbell narrow squats

four sets of twelve shoulder-width hack squat

Tuesday

Superset

four sets of twelve side lateral raise

four sets of twelve seated barbell press

four sets of high rope pull

Superset

four sets of fifteen pushdowns

four sets of fifteen overhead presses

four sets of twelve bench dips

Wednesday

six sets of twelve wide-grip pulldowns

Superset

four sets of fifteen cable rows

four sets of fifteen one-arm dumbbell row

Superset

five sets of twelve incline dumbbell curl

five sets of twelve seated dumbbell curl

Thursday

Superset

five sets of fifteen leg curls

five sets of fifteen weighted bench step up

Superset

five sets of twelve seated leg curl

five sets of fifteen stiff leg

five sets of sumo dumbbell squat, but rest for 30 seconds before beginning each set

Friday

Superset

four sets of twelve incline fly

four sets of ten incline presses

Superset

four sets of fifteen on the butt machine

four sets of fifteen on the stability ball with your butt raised

Superset

Four sets of fifteen weighted sumo squats

four sets of fifteen cable butt kick backs

Workout Three

Monday

Superset

Four sets of fifteen leg extensions

four sets of ten narrow dumbbell squats

Superset

four sets of twenty shoulder width leg presses

four sets of fifteen switch jumping lunge

four sets of fifteen narrow stance using the smith machine squats

Tuesday

Superset

four sets of ten barbell shoulder presses

four sets of ten wide-grip overhead barbell raise

four sets of ten rear lateral raise

six sets of eight lateral side raise, but rest for twenty second before starting the next set

Superset

three sets of fifteen rope pushdowns

three sets of ten dumbbell nose crushers

three sets of fifteen dumbbell kick backs

Wednesday

four sets of eight wide-grip pull downs

four sets of eight seated close-grip cable row

Superset

four sets of twelve palms up reverse-grip barbell rows

four sets of twelve assisted pull ups

five sets of fifteen hyperextensions

Superset

four sets of eight preacher curls

four sets of twelve seated dumbbell curl

four sets of incline fifteen dumbbell curls

Thursday

Superset

four sets of fifteen leg curls

five sets of twelve leg presses

Superset

Five sets of twelve seated leg curls

five sets of twelve stiff legs

Friday

Superset

five sets of twelve flat fly

five sets of twelve incline cheer press

Superset

five sets of fifteen wide machine smith squat

five sets of bosu ball squat

Superset

four sets of twenty hyperextensions

four sets of on the butt machine

Chapter 5. Additional Tips

The cardio sessions are really tailored to be tough and do not become discouraged if you are not able to complete everything for the first time. You can try harder the next day and also the next until you become really better. It can take more than a week to build endurance so you can complete a whole session. You know that you have worked really hard if your body is sore the next day.

You can follow this training plan and ask your trainer to design a cardio and weight lifting routine that is appropriate for you. You can start with light impact exercises and gradually increase the impact as you progress. An example of a good cardio workout is running on a treadmill with increasing and decreasing incline alternately which can be a form of interval training that helps in building endurance and stamina. You can also do sprints with jogging for 30 seconds in between.

For the weight training, you should not do more than one weight training session in one day. You can breakup your training for morning and night. You can do the weight training in the morning and then the cardio at night. In case you should do them both consecutively, you should always do the weight training first. You should also follow a diet plan for your training to get the best results and you need to stay energized throughout your cardio and weight training sessions.

Conclusion

Weight lifting for women has become more popular and it is no longer only for men. Women who really get into weight lifting join competitions locally internationally. They follow a very strict diet that is rich in protein and foods that are god for building muscle. Proper diet is very important because it takes a great amount of energy to be lifting weights. Compound exercises are usually focused on so you will work the proper muscle groups for you to be able to lift weights. You also need to take note of the principles mentioned in this book because they give a very detailed explanation on how sessions should be performed for you to effectively target and work your muscles.

A good range of motion is important because it is more effective than doing incomplete ranges of motion in multiple exercises. Remember that it is more of the quality of the movements that you are doing compared to the number of exercises done with less effort. It will help in building your endurance and strength fast. You also need to be aware of the muscle groups that you work each day because there is a recovery time that your muscles require in order to rebuild. Do not over train your body and at the same time do not work the same muscle groups for two days in a row because you will not allow them to recover. If you do not allow them to recover, your muscles will not rebuild and it will take longer for you to build muscles. If you want them to build faster, proper diet and training session should be observed.

You should also be aware of your body fat because you may need to do more to get rid of your body fat, but always consult your doctor if you are safe to do weight lifting. Your trainer will be able to give you the proper training plan, but your doctor will tell if it is safe for you to do this. You should not get discouraged if you need to try harder for your fitness to build up because all people start from somewhere and they will not be where they are today if they did not undergo the process of progressing over time as they practice harder each day. All you need is motivation, inspiration, and determination because without these 3, you will not have the proper mindset to continue with your training until you become a lot better than when you first started. You should also not be ashamed if you are a beginner because everyone was once a beginner and they also had to try harder to get to where they are today.

If you are just starting out, you can get tips from this book and take note of the foods that you need to eat so that you will be prepared for anything that your trainer will make you do. Pushing your body is a good way to strengthen your immune system, but you also need the proper diet to support yourself. Do not let anything stop you because everyone goes through challenges and you need those so that you will become stronger.

Thank You Page

I want to personally thank you for reading my book. I hope you found information in this book useful and I would be very grateful if you could leave your honest review about this book. I certainly want to thank you in advance for doing this.

If you have the time, you can check my other books too.

www.ingramcontent.com/pod-product-compliance
Lightning Source LLC
LaVergne TN
LVHW021743060526
838200LV00052B/3437